The 2 Day Diet: 5:2 Diet

70 Top Recipes & Cookbook
To Lose Weight & Sustain It
Now Revealed!

(Fasting Day Edition)

Table of Contents

Introduction

Today, there are a growing number of overweight and obese people in the world. According to the WHO, over 500 million people in the world are already considered as obese. This is an alarming number because over 65% of these people live in countries where obesity is a major cause of morbidity. Furthermore, obese and overweight people are prone to illnesses and health risks such as stroke and heart attack. This is why going on a diet and regular exercising is necessary.

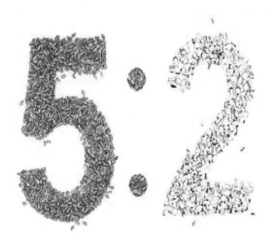

While there are many forms of diet currently available, many of them will not work for you. This is because most of them force you to go on a drastic diet that will result in lack of energy and increase food cravings. Such diets can also be detrimental to your health. If you want something that can really help you lose weight without suppressing most cravings, the 5:2 Diet may be a great idea for you.

What is the 5:2 Diet?

This diet limits the calorie intake of people in two days (called the fasting days) and eating normal on the remaining 5 days of the week.

Basis Of The Diet

The general idea of this diet is to let you fast and go on a calorie-restricted diet for two given days within a week and the other remaining 5 days you eat as you normally do. This does not require a full fasting as in you take only water for two days. No. What it requires you to do is limit and keeps your calorie intake at a minimum for two days. The two fasting days should also not be consecutive as doing it consecutively will result in cravings. This diet is said to help lose weight in as little as one month, decrease cholesterol levels and blood sugar levels.

Choosing The Days For Fasting

It is actually up to you when you want to go fasting. You can go fasting on Monday and Thursday or Tuesday and Friday. It depends on when is most convenient for you. It is generally not advised to go on fasting two consecutive days as hunger pangs become stronger the longer you go fasting. But if this is most convenient for you, it is still okay provided that you don't exceed 48 hours of fasting. Also, it is best to talk to your physician if you intend to go on 2 consecutive days fasting.

What You Should Eat And When

There is really no restriction to what you want to eat. You can eat whatever you like as long as you don't exceed the required calorie intake. Men are required to limit calorie intake for 600 calories and for women 500 calories. When you want to eat is also dependent on you. If you have breakfast at 10am or 5am, it doesn't really matter. What is most important with this diet is adhering to the required calorie intake on fast days. What you want to eat and when you want to eat is dependent on you.

How to Shop for Food and How to Dine Out

When it comes to shopping for food, it is advised that you always read the label. Check how much calories is one serving of the food that you eat before you buy to make sure that you don't exceed the required calorie intake. Also, it can be very helpful if you already have a meal for the week planned so you know how what you need to buy and how much calories each of the items you need to get are. This will help you save time when shopping for food.

When it comes to dining out, it is best that you do it on feast days instead. During your fasting days, eat food you prepared or bought instead so you don't go beyond the calorie limit. Of course, when eating at a restaurant you certainly wouldn't want to restrict yourself with eating the delectable meals they offer, would you? So, it is best that you schedule dining out on your feast days. Don't worry because the 5:2 Diet is actually very flexible and you can always interchange the days when you want to fast and days when you want to feast.

70 Top Recipes to Try

Breakfast Recipes

Breakfast is said to be the most important meal of the day. It is true, actually because this is the meal that powers our body to accomplish tasks for the day. But that does not mean you need to eat foods high in calories to suffice your daily energy needs. These recipes of the 5:2 Diet will attest that though breakfast is important it should not consist of too much calories.

Greek yogurt

Yogurt is a great breakfast food because it contains high amounts of protein and good bacteria that can supply your daily energy needs. Best of all, it only contains 48 calories.

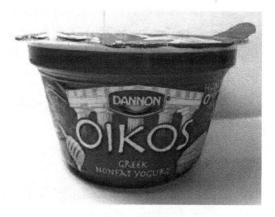

Banana, apple, or oranges

Fruits contain fructose which is a good source of sugar to convert into energy. Fruits are also rich in fiber and very low on calories. Banana only has 90 calories, apples have 53 calories, and oranges have 59 calories.

Boiled egg

Egg is a staple breakfast food. If you want this for breakfast, stay away from omelet, sunny side up, or scrambled eggs. Eat boiled eggs instead as these are low in calories with only 89 calories. You can go for soft boiled (boil for 3 minutes), medium boiled (boiled for 5 minutes), or hard boiled (boiled for 10 minutes or even more).

2 slices of Ryvita crisp breads

Eating bread alone can suffice your breakfast needs. 2 slices of Ryvita crisp breads has only 64 calories - perfect for your fasting days.

Baked beans

Beans contain high amounts of protein and low in saturated fat making it a great meal to start your day with. One can of Heinz baked beans contain only 100 calories and are enough to keep your tummy satisfied until lunch time.

Pea smoothie

This is a delicious and refreshing breakfast drink that is sure to keep you satisfied but at the same time maintain your desired calorie intake for the day as it only contains 190 calories per serving.

Ingredients:
- 1 bag of raw frozen peas
- 1 cup organic strawberries
- ½ cup fresh pineapple juice
- 1 medium-sized banana sliced

Procedure:
- Cook peas as directed by the manufacturer. Rinse with cold water after until completely cooled.
- Blend 1/3 of the cooked peas with all the other ingredients until thick and smooth.
- Reserve remaining peas for tomorrow.

Recipe serves 2 glasses.

Crumpets

These are low on calories (only 100 calories) and very easy to make on your own. Serve this with sugar-free fruit jam or low fat butter.

Ingredients:
- 350ml warm skimmed milk
- 450g all purpose flour or whole wheat flour
- 5g dried yeast
- 2 teaspoons of granulated sugar
- 350ml warm water
- 1 tsp iodized salt
- 1tsp baking powder
- A little drizzle of vegetable or olive oil for cooking

Procedure:
- On one bowl whisk together milk, flour, sugar, and yeast. Whisk just until combined.
- Add half of the water to the mixture. Continue adding water until you reach a thick and smooth batter. Do not add more if the consistency already resembles a thick cream.
- Cover it with a plastic wrap and place in a draft-free area for 1-2 hours to foam.
- After said time, whisk in yeast and baking powder.
- Heat up a pan on a stove. Make sure it is hot but not smoking hot.
- Grease the base of the pan with vegetable oil and place crumpet rings.
- Place the batter inside the ring and cook for about 5 minutes. There should be many tiny holes on top and the crumpet is already set.
- Flip the crumpet and cook on the other side for another 2 minutes.
- Once done, serve and enjoy eating.

Brown bread

A slice of brown bread for breakfast is another great food to eat. This is rich in fiber and has only 74 calories per slice.

Egg white omelets

If you really must have eggs but don't want boiled eggs, you can eat egg white omelets. Remove the egg yolks of 2 eggs and fry only the eggs whites. This has only 34 calories. Eat it with crumpets and you only gain 134 calories. Or, eat it with brown bread and gain only 108 calories.

Poached egg with ham

If you want something heavier and fuller on your stomach, this is a great idea to have for breakfast. Poached egg with one slice of ham combined only has 100 calories.

Lunch Recipes

Lunch is probably the heaviest of all meals that people usually take. With lunch, you have the excuse to eat more than for dinner and eat more delectable meals than for breakfast. But that is also not a reason to binge on too much calories. The recipes and foods below will allow you to eat good food but with lesser amount of calories.

Miso soup

Miso soup is a great way to enjoy a hot meal for lunch without packing on the calories. One sachet of the Itsu miso soup has only 44 calories.

Carrot and lentil Soup

Heinz carrot and lentil soup has only 87 calories per serving making it a great dish for lunch especially on colder months.

Tomato soup

Another soup by Heinz is their tomato soup that has only 76 calories.

Cauliflower with low-fat cheese

Cauliflower is not only rich in vitamins and minerals but is also rich in fiber while at the same time has only 23 calories per 87g. Non-fat mozzarella cheese adds some flavor to this recipe and 50g of it has only 70.5 calories.

Ingredients:
- 174g of cauliflower
- 50g or non-fat mozzarella cheese
- Some salt and pepper
- Freshly chopped parsley for garnish

Procedure:
- Cook cauliflower on boiling water.
- Drain and place on a baking dish.
- Add mozzarella cheese on top and sprinkle with some salt and pepper.

- Bake just until cheese melts.
- Top with chopped parsley and serve.

Flatbread with tomato garlic sauce and anchovies

This is a savory lunch meal that is also low in calories (only 224).

- Ingredients:
- ½ tsp of olive oil
- 1 garlic clove peeled and minced
- 1tbsp tomato paste or puree
- 4 pieces anchovy fillets
- 1 piece Flatbread

Procedure:
- In a small frying pan, pour olive oil and heat for a few seconds.
- Add garlic and brown for about 1-2 minutes.
- Stir in tomato paste or puree and add 2 tbsp of water and fry slightly for 4-5 minutes.
- Spread the tomato sauce on a flatbread and top with anchovy fillets.

Baked apple

This recipe has only 185 calories.

Ingredients:
- 1 piece of large Bramley apple
- 1 tsp of low-fat butter
- 5g of slivered almonds
- 2 tsp dark brown sugar
- ½ tsp of mixed spices, grounded
- 10g of raisins
- Orange zest (half an orange)

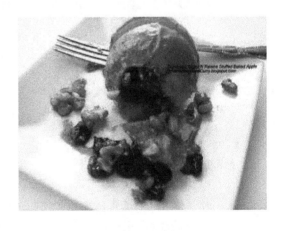

Procedure:
- Preheat oven to 190 degrees C.
- Core the apple and using a scorer, score the middle.
- Mix all the other ingredients in a small bowl (to be used as filling).

- Stuff the apple with the filling. If there are still some left, rub the outsides of the apple as well.
- Place the apple on a baking dish and bake for about 35-40 minutes – just until golden in color and soft.

Chicken Satay

Chicken contains lesser amount of calories and fat making it a great meal for the 5:2 Diet. This recipe has only 244 calories.

Ingredients:
- 250g cubed chicken breasts
- 1 piece shallots sliced and peeled
- 1 clove of garlic peeled and minced
- 2 tsp curry powder
- 1 tbsp of peanut butter
- 1 tsp of raw honey
- 2 tbsp soy sauce

Procedure:
- Mix shallots, garlic, curry powder, honey, peanut butter and soy sauce in a mixing bowl.
- Toss in the chicken and massage the marinade to the chicken to absorb it well.
- Marinade the chicken for 3-4 hours inside the refrigerator.
- Once done, you can either grill it or bake it.

Halloumi Salad

Salads are definitely the easiest dishes to create that are sure to be low in calories and high in fiber. This recipe only has 215 calories.

Ingredients:
- 2 pieces of ripe tomatoes
- ½ red bell pepper seeded and cut into long strips
- 50g of light halloumi sliced into thin strips or squares and drained
- 75g of various Italian greens
- ½ clove of garlic peeled and minced

- 1 lime juice
- 1 tsp parsley freshly chopped
- ½ tsp of red pepper flakes
- Some freshly ground black pepper
- 1 tsp of olive oil

Procedure:

- In a mixing bowl, combine garlic, parsley, lime juice, black pepper, pepper flakes, olive oil and 1tbsp of water. Add some sliced tomatoes.
- In a large frying pan, heat the oil and fry the red bell peppers until dry for 5 minutes. Add them to the mixture.
- Add the halloumi and marinade it for a few hours. Make sure all parts are coated with the marinade.
- On a serving plate, arrange the greens. Add the halloumi on top, some tomatoes and sliced bell peppers. Drizzle with some marinade and serve.

Tuna salad

Another great recipe to eat for lunch is tuna salad. Not only is this very easy to make but also has only 178 calories.

Ingredients:
- 350g tuna flakes
- 3tbsp soy sauce
- 1tsp horseradish or wasabi
- 1tbsp white wine or sake
- 200g various greens
- 150g yellow tomatoes cut in half
- 1 cucumber sliced into strips
- 2tbsp soy sauce
- 1tbsp lime or lemon juice
- 1tbsp brown or muscovado sugar
- 1tsp sesame or olive oil

Procedure:

- Combine first four ingredients in a mixing bowl and marinade for about 10 minutes.
- Arrange greens, cucumber, and tomatoes on a plate
- Combine last 4 ingredients on a separate mixing bowl (dressing).
- Heat a frying pan on high and fry the tuna flakes until cooked.
- Place tuna on top of arrange vegetables and drizzle with salad dressing.

Apple and blackberry muffins

This is a complete meal containing carbohydrates, protein, and vitamins. One piece contains 200 calories.

Ingredients:
- 6tbsp of muscovado or brown sugar
- 1 apple, preferably red apple sliced and cored
- 200g chopped blackberries
- 1tsp cinnamon, grounded
- 250g whole meal or whole wheat flour
- 4tsp baking powder
- 2 beaten eggs
- 125ml skimmed milk
- 125ml grape seed oil for cooking

Procedure:
- In a mixing bowl, mix together apple, blackberries, cinnamon, and sugar. Set aside.
- On a separate bowl, sift together flour and baking powder.
- Create a hole in the middle.
- On a separate bowl, mix together milk, oil, and eggs. Pour the mixture into the hole created on the dry ingredients.
- Stir the dry and wet ingredients just until combined.
- Fold in fruit mixture.
- Pour mixture into muffin liners lined pan and bake for 20-30 minutes at 200 degrees C.

Mushroom Stroganoff

This is definitely delicious meal has only 90 calories.

Ingredients:
- 1 tbsp grape seed oil for cooking
- 1 sliced and peeled onion
- 4 sticks of celery sliced thinly
- 2 garlic cloves peeled and minced
- 600g or various mushrooms (button, shitake, etc)
- 2tsp of paprika, smoked variant
- 250ml vegetable stock
- 150ml yogurt or sour cream
- A dash of pepper

Procedure:
- In a non-stick pan, heat oil. Toss in onions, celery and then garlic and cook for about 5 minutes –just until soft.
- Add in the mushrooms and sprinkle with paprika and cook for another 5 minutes.
- Pour in the vegetable stock and continue boiling until the liquid is reduced into half.
- Pour in yogurt or sour cream and sprinkle with a dash of pepper.
- Cook over medium heat for a few more minutes.
- Serve immediately.

Hash corned beef

If you really want meat for lunch, this is a great recipe to try that has only 227 calories.

Ingredients:
- 1tsp vegetable or olive oil
- 1 piece onion, peeled and chopped
- 350g of cooked potatoes, peeled and chopped
- 300g can of corned beef
- 1tbsp freshly chopped parsley

- Some Worcestershire sauce
- A dash of salt and pepper

Procedure:
- In a large frying pan, heat oil. Add in the onions and cook until translucent (about 5 minutes).
- Toss in the potatoes and corned beef and cook for another 7 minutes mixing them occasionally.
- Toss in the parsley and add the Worcestershire sauce, salt, and pepper.
- Serve immediately.

Chicken salsa burger

This is a healthy and low-calorie twist to the all-time favorite burger. This recipe has only 135 calories.

Ingredients:
- 1 crushed clove of garlic
- 3 finely chopped spring onions
- 1 tbsp of pesto sauce
- 2 tbsp of various herbs such as tarragon, parsley, thyme and rosemary
- 375g of minced chicken flesh
- 2 pieces of tomatoes, sun dried
- 1 tsp olive oil
- 250g of quartered cherry tomatoes
- 1 piece of seeded and chopped red chili pepper
- 1 tbsp of chopped coriander
- 1 lime zest and juice

Procedure:
- In a mixing bowl, combine first 6 ingredients.
- Divide the mixture into 4 equal parts and shape them into round balls before flattening them.
- In a separate bowl, mix together last 4 ingredients.
- Lightly brush a frying pan or griller with olive oil.

- Place flattened burger patties on the grill or pan and cook on each side about 2-4 minutes.
- Serve together with the salsa and enjoy.

Mushrooms and whole meal toast

If you prefer something light, this is a great idea. This has only 110 calories but is sure to be tasty as well.

Ingredients:
- 100g mushrooms
- 2 slices Whole meal bread
- Low-fat butter or olive oil
- Dash of salt and pepper

Procedure:
- Cook mushrooms on low-fat butter or olive oil for a few minutes until soft and tender.
- Sprinkle with some salt and pepper.
- Top on your whole meal bread and enjoy.

Smoke salmon and wheat crackers

This meal has only 48 calories.
- Ingredients:
- Salmon
- Salt and pepper
- Olive oil
- Wheat crackers

Procedure:
- Rub salt and pepper to salmon on both sides.
- Coat the griller with olive oil and grill the salmon.
- Brush it with olive oil as you cook it to prevent drying.
- Once done, serve with whole wheat crackers and enjoy.

Fruit bowl

You can have a bowl of various fruits to give you enough energy while at the same time keeps your calorie intake at a minimum. This combination of fruits has only 178 calories.

Ingredients:
- 100g lychees
- 100g cherries
- 1 nectarine

Roasted pepper with feta cheese

This recipe has only 130 calories.

Ingredients:
- Green and red bell peppers
- Oil
- Slices of feta cheese

Procedure:
- Brush the griller with some olive oil and roast bell peppers on both sides. Don't forget to brush the peppers with olive oil as you grill them to prevent drying.
- Serve with feta cheese on the side.

Toasted bread with creamy mushroom and garlic

This recipe is so delicious you wouldn't even think it has only 190 calories.

Ingredients:
- 100g of mushrooms
- low-fat butter
- 3 cloves of garlic peeled and minced
- Low-fat cream cheese
- Whole meal bread

Procedure:

- Heat a frying pan with butter and sauté garlic and mushroom until golden brown and soft. Add cream cheese. Mix until cheese melts.
- Spread some butter on bread and toast it. Top it with garlic, mushroom, and cream cheese mixture and enjoy.

Baguette and cheese

This is a very simple meal that is light and satisfying but has only 151 calories.

Ingredients:

- One small slice of baguette
- 50g of non-fat mozzarella cheese

Procedure:

- Place cheese on top of baguette and bake until cheese melts.
- Once done, top with some parsley and serve.

Allotment soup with croutons

This is the perfect meal for colder days. It has only 105 calories.

Ingredients:

- Olive oil for cooking
- 300g of various peppers (red, green, and yellow)
- 400g of diced tomatoes
- 2 small courgettes, finely chopped
- 2 medium-sized onions, skinned and finely chopped
- 2 medium-sized carrots, skinned and chopped
- 4 cloves of garlic, peeled and minced
- 400ml of vegetable stock
- ½ tsp of paprika, smoked version
- A dash of salt and pepper

Procedure:

- Drizzle olive oil on frying pan and fry all the vegetables in the recipe.
- Cover the pan and let the vegetables cook for 5minutes over high heat.
- Pour in vegetable stock and sprinkle with smoked paprika, salt, and pepper.
- Simmer for about 45 minutes over low heat.
- Cool slightly and transfer half of the mixture to a blender.
- Puree the mixture then pour the mixture back to the pan.
- Reheat the soup and add more salt and pepper if needed.
- Serve with freshly chopped parsley and some croutons on top.

Salmon and herb fishcakes

This is a very tasty treat that has only 285 calories.

Ingredients:
- 200g salmon
- 140g mashed potatoes
- 1tbsp chives, freshly chopped
- 1tbsp parsley, freshly chopped
- 1tsp capers, chopped and drained
- 1tsp Tabasco or hot sauce
- A dash of salt and pepper
- 1tbsp all purpose flour
- Olive oil for frying

Procedure:
- Mash the salmon flesh and discard skin.
- In a mixing bowl, combine the mashed salmon flesh with mashed potatoes, chives, parsley and capers. Add Tabasco or hot sauce and sprinkle with some salt and pepper.
- On a lightly floured surface, roll the mixture into a sausage shape and wrap in cling wrap and chill inside the freezer for 30 minutes.
- When you are all ready to cook, slice the fish cakes and dust with some flour.
- Drizzle pan with olive oil and cook fish cakes on both sides until golden brown in color.

- Serve with green salad and enjoy.

Bacon, wine, and risotto

This is a great recipe for the holidays or any special occasion but it has only 380 calories.

Ingredients;
- 2 rashers of lean bacon
- 100g chopped mushrooms
- 2 pieces of dried porcini mushroom
- Vegetable oil or olive oil for cooking
- Medium onion peeled and sliced
- 175g risotto
- 150ml dry white wine
- 300ml vegetable stock
- Parsley
- A dash of salt and pepper

Procedure:
- Grill bacon until golden brown and crispy then chop into small pieces.
- Drizzle a frying pan with oil and sauté mushrooms until soft (about 5 minutes) then season with salt and pepper.
- Add porcini mushrooms to sautéed mushrooms. Fry them until soft.
- Add the rice, wine, and soaking water of the porcini mushrooms to the mixture and stir them all together vigorously.
- Stir in the bacon and add the vegetable stock.
- Transfer the mixture to a baking dish.
- Cover with aluminum foil and bake for 25-30 minutes in 200 degrees C.

Roasted red bell pepper soup

Not only is red bell pepper rich in vitamin C, it is also low in calories. This soup recipe has only 100 calories per serving.

Ingredients:
- 4 large red bell peppers seeded and chopped
- Olive oil
- 2 medium-sized onions skinned and finely chopped
- 1 tbsp of fennel seeds
- 4 garlic closed peeled and minced
- 1 small red chili pepper diced
- 400g tomatoes
- 1200ml vegetable stock
- 2-3 dashes of Tabasco or hot sauce
- A dash of salt and pepper
- Fresh basil for garnish

Procedure:
- Grill red bell peppers until charred. Once done, place in a plastic bag to cool. Once cooled, peel skin off and finely chop the flesh.
- Pour olive oil in a frying pan and sauté onions and fennel seeds over medium heat for 5 minutes.
- Add the flesh of red bell peppers and all the other ingredients except for basil.
- Bring mixture to a boil and then reduce heat and let simmer for 15-20 minutes.
- Pour mixture to a blender and blend until smooth.
- Sprinkle with more salt and pepper if needed. Serve with toasted bread and garnish with basil.

Cauliflower pizza

This is a healthy and low-calorie twist to pizza with only 240 calories per serving (recipe can serve 2 people).

Ingredients:
- 340g fresh cauliflower
- 1 free range egg, large size
- 75g non-fat or low fat mozzarella cheese
- 2tbsp of parmesan cheese
- ¼ tsp dried basil leaves

- ¼ tsp dried oregano
- ¼ tsp garlic powder
- Sea or rock salt
- Freshly grounded black pepper
- 2 fresh and raw tomatoes sliced thinly
- ½ medium sized red onion skinned and sliced thinly
- 2 cloves of garlic peeled and minced
- ¼ tsp of red chili powder or flakes
- Fresh oregano or basil (for garnish only)

Procedure:
- Grate cauliflower or process in a food processor until crumbly – not pureed.
- Pop the cauliflower crumbs inside the microwave for 5-6minutes very soft. You can also boil it instead but make sure to squeeze out excess water once cooked.
- Place cooked cauliflower crumbs in a mixing bowl and add grated mozzarella cheese (50g of the recipe), all the herbs, parmesan cheese, and egg, salt, pepper, and garlic powder. Mix them all well until dough forms.
- Shape dough into a ball and pat it flat on a baking tray lined with parchment paper. Spray the top of the dough with a little oil and bake for 15-20 minutes in 210 degrees C until golden brown.
- Top the baked dough with tomato slices, minced garlic, some onion rings, chili flakes and sprinkle with some salt and pepper. Put 25g of mozzarella cheese slices on top and bake again just until cheese melts.
- Garnish with basil and serve.

Dinner Recipes

If you are on a diet, you know for a fact that you shouldn't eat too much during dinnertime. This is the time of the day when our metabolism is the slowest and therefore, eating too much will result in stored calories which will eventually turn into fat. The recipes and foods listed below will help you have a great dinner while at the same time maintain your desired calorie intake for the day.

Grilled chicken breast

This recipe has only 162 calories.

Ingredients:
- 150g chicken breast
- A dash of salt and pepper
- Olive oil

Procedure:
- Rub salt and pepper on both sides of the chicken.
- Brush the griller with olive oil. Once hot, grill chicken on both sides brushing with olive oil as you cook to prevent drying.
- Serve with cherry tomatoes if you prefer.

Chili Chicken Noodle Salad by Tesco

This can be found in most groceries and has only 195 calories.

Cod Steak with Parsley Sauce by Young

This is also available in most groceries and one serving has only 101 calories.

Cod with Noodles Asian Style by Marks and Spencer

This is another great meal that can easily be bought at most M&S stores perfect for busy people who don't have time to cook. This has only 215 calories.

Cooked peas

Peas are also a great source of vitamins and protein and 38g can/bag of this has only 38 calories.

Prawns

If you want something special for dinner, cooked prawns is a great idea. 50g of this has only 40 calories.

Ingredients:
- 50g prawns
- Dash of salt and pepper
- Olive oil

Procedure:
- Heat frying pan and drizzle with olive oil.
- Once hot (but not smoking hot) fry the prawns.
- Sprinkle with some salt and pepper and wait for the prawns to turn into orange.

Asparagus

It may be one of the most expensive vegetables but it is definitely one of the healthiest as well. 10 spears of this contain only 50 calories. This recipe has only 88 calories.

Ingredients:
- 10 spears of asparagus
- 2tbsp low-fat mayonnaise
- Salt and pepper
- 2 cloves Minced garlic

Procedure:
- Steam asparagus spears until cooked
- In a mixing bowl, mix mayonnaise, salt, pepper, and garlic to make the dip.
- Dip cooked asparagus spears on the garlic-mayo dip and enjoy.

Salmon fillet

Seafood is definitely a great food to have a satisfying meal while at the same time maintain a low calorie intake. Half fillet of salmon has only 185 calories.

Ingredients:
- One half fillet salmon
- Olive oil
- Salt and pepper

Procedure:
- Rub salt and pepper on both sides of salmon fillet.
- Brush griller with olive oil.
- Once hot, grill salmon fillet on both sides.
- Brush the salmon with some olive oil as you cook to prevent drying.
- Serve with cauliflower if desired.

Asparagus and prosciutto frittata

If you want something delectable while at the same time maintain your diet this is a great recipe to try. This has only 125 calories.

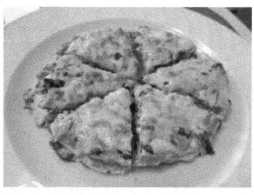

Ingredients:
- 2 medium-sized eggs
- 125g asparagus
- 2 slices of prosciutto
- 40g of peeled red onions sliced thinly
- Some olive oil or vegetable oil for cooking

Procedure:
- Steam asparagus until cooked and wash with cold water.
- Heat a frying pan and drizzle with oil.
- Sauté onions and prosciutto. When onions are translucent in color, add in the asparagus.
- In a bowl, beat eggs thoroughly and pour into pan to coat the other ingredients.
- Once bottom has cooked, flip eggs over and cook the other side.
- Serve with tomato salad if desired.

Summer salad

This is a very refreshing salad perfect for the summertime; it has only 147 calories.

Ingredients:
- 60g of watercress
- 100g of various radishes sliced finely
- 10g of peeled and thinly sliced red onion
- 90g of diced waitrose sweetfire beetroot
- 1tsp low-fat mayonnaise
- 1tsp horseradish or wasabi paste
- 2tsp 0%fat Greek yogurt
- Freshly chopped parsley for garnish

Procedure:
- Spread chopped watercress on a serving plate.
- Scatter various radishes, onions, and beetroot on top of the watercress.
- In a mixing bowl, mix wasabi or horseradish, mayonnaise, parsley, and yogurt.
- Drizzle the sauce on top of the salad and serve.

Calamari and Greek salad

This is another salad recipe you can enjoy for your dinner. This salad has only 281 calories.

Ingredients:
- ½ bag of calamari rings
- 30g hummus
- ½ bag of various greens
- 65g of olives and feta cheese
- 40g sliced cucumber
- 65g sliced cherry tomatoes

Procedure:
- Arrange greens on a serving plate.

- Top it with cucumber, cherry tomatoes, calamari rings, olives and feta cheese.
- Spoon dollops of hummus and serve.

Smoked salmon and pita bread

This recipe has only 195 calories.

Ingredients:
- 1 white pita bread
- 1tbsp low-fat cream cheese
- 25g smoked salmon slices
- ¼ of medium red onion skinned and diced
- 1tsp of capers
- 40g lettuce
- dill
- 1 wedge of lemon

Procedure:
- Spread cream cheese on pita bread.
- Arrange on top salmon slices, lettuce, capers, dill and red onions.
- Bake until cheese melts for 180 degrees C.
- Serve with lemon wedge on the side.

Baked chicken breasts with herbs and spices

This recipe has only 190 calories per serving.

Ingredients:
- 2 150g chicken breast slices
- Parsley, oregano or basil
- 1/4tsp cumin, ground
- 1/4tsp coriander, ground
- Olive oil
- 250ml or 1 can vegetable stock
- Dash of salt, pepper, and chili powder to taste

Procedure:

- Rub all herbs, salt, pepper, and chili powder to chicken on both sides. Make sure it is evenly coated.
- Transfer on a baking dish and pour in vegetable stock.
- Bake for 20-25 minutes at 200 degrees C.
- Serve with salad if desired.

Scallops with leeks and pancetta

This recipe has only 247 calories.

Ingredients:

- 2 8g thin slices of bacon or pancetta
- 85g medium scallops
- 50g leeks, washed and sliced
- 80g fresh peas
- Six fronds of dill or sprigs
- 30g leaves of wild rocket

Procedure:

- Fry the pancetta or bacon until crispy and fat is drained.
- On a serving plate arrange scallops, leeks, peas, sprigs, and wild rocket.
- Toss in cooked pancetta and serve.

Cheese and tomato omelet

This recipe has only 170 calories.

Ingredients:

- Olive oil or grape seed oil for cooking
- 35g halved cherry tomatoes
- ¼ of medium sized red onions skinned and diced
- 6-8 leaves of fresh basil finely chopped
- 2 free range eggs, small
- 1tbsp parmesan cheese, grated
- A dash of pepper and salt

Procedure:

- Heat a frying pan with olive oil.
- Sauté onions until soft and translucent in color. Add in cherry tomatoes and cook until juices are released.
- In a mixing bowl, beat the eggs thoroughly.
- Pour the beaten eggs into the frying pan. Sprinkle with salt, pepper, parmesan cheese, and basil.
- Once bottom is cooked flip over to cook the other side.
- Serve with toasted whole meal bread if desired.

Fridge salad

This salad has only 230 calories.

Ingredients:

- 40g mixed greens
- 1 peeled and chopped small carrot
- 2 sliced spring onions
- 3 halved cherry tomatoes
- 8 cucumber slices
- 50g quartered pickled beets
- 38g broken into pieces feta cheese
- 1tbsp balsamic vinegar
- A dash of black pepper

Procedure:

- In a mixing bowl, toss first 7 ingredients.
- Mix in balsamic vinegar and sprinkle with black pepper.

Light Snacks

In case you feel hungry in between meals, there are snacks you can try that are also very low on calories but enough to keep you satisfied until your next meal.

- Apples and yogurt Rhis snack recipe has only 45 calories.

    ○ Core ½ apple and bake until soft.
    ○ Top with 1tbsp low-fat yogurt and sprinkle with some cinnamon.

- ½ frozen small bananas contain only 45 calories.

- One miniature box of raisins is also a great snack containing only 45 calories.

- Cherries are also a great snack and 12 pieces of them has only 48 calories.

- Combine 2 ½ tbsps. of 0% fat Greek yogurt and ½ cup of strawberries and you only gain 47 calories.

- 14 frozen seedless grapes only have 48 calories.

- 1 rod of pretzels only has 37 calories.
    ○
- ½ cup of edamame without shells and sprinkled with sea salt only has 37 calories.

- Slice one medium-sized cucumber and mix it with ¼ cup of diced onions, ½ cup of finely chopped celery, 4tbsp of vinegar and sprinkle with some salt. This snack only has 45 calories.

- One small stalk of celery with ½ tbsp of peanut butter only has 49 calories.

- One brown rice cake served with 1tbsp of any sugar-free jam only has 44 calories.

- Cucumber slices with low-fat garlic and herbs cheese dip only has 35 calories.

- 8 grape-sized tomatoes with 1tbsp of low-fat cream cheese only have 46 calories.

- Broil 1 large tomato topped with 1tbsp of grated parmesan cheese contains 44 calories.

- 1 ounce of fat-free mozzarella cheese with 1tsp marinara sauce dip only has 46 calories.

- 2 slices of grilled turkey meat wrapped in lettuce only has 46 calories.

- 1 ounce of smoked salmon placed on top of wheat crackers only has 48 calories.

- 1.3 ounces of tuna flakes with a teaspoon of Dijon mustard spread on wheat crackers only has about 60 calories.

- 1 slice of crisp wheat bread with 2tsps of hummus on top has 45 calories.

- Half of a small grapefruit only has 32 calories.

Bonus Section

500-Calorie Meal Plan on Fasting Days

Meal Plan 1:

Breakfast – banana (90 calories) and two pieces of crackers (34 calories)
Lunch – beetroot and cheese salad (172 calories)
Dinner – chicken tikka masala (200 calories)
Total: 496 calories

Meal Plan 2:

Breakfast: hardboiled egg served with Satsuma (103 calories)
Lunch: Mediterranean Veg Quiche from Weight Watchers and side salad from Tesco (178 calories)
Dinner: leek soup with cheese toasts (200 calories)
Total: 481 calories

Meal Plan 3:

Breakfast: banana milkshake using ½ banana, 6 ounces skim milk, 1tsp of pure vanilla extract, 1/3 cup crushed ice blended all together in a blender and topped with tangerine wedge (152 calories)
Lunch: Creamy Vegetable Soup by Sainsbury with rice cake (88 calories).
Dinner: beef stew (240 calories)
Total: 480 calories

Meal Plan 3:

Breakfast: fruit and nut bar by Alpen with crackers from Tuc (133 calories)
Lunch: toasted rye bread with baked beans (195 calories)
Dinner: low-fat prawn tom yum soup (172 calories)
Total: 500 calories

Meal Plan 4:

Breakfast: white chocolate and strawberry cereal bar from Tesco (85 calories)
Lunch: Chicken Noodle Salad with Chili from Tesco (195 calories)
Dinner: vegetable balti curry (211 calories)
Total: 491 calories

600-Calorie Meal Plans

Meal Plan 1:

Breakfast: steel cut oats with ½ cup fresh blueberries (190 calories)
Lunch: roasted red bell pepper soup (100 calories)
Dinner: stir-fried chicken with 1 tangerine (306 calories)
Total: 596 calories

Meal Plan 2:

Breakfast: smoked salmon with Ryvita crackers and low-fat cream cheese (178 calories)
Lunch: fried prawns (40 calories)
Dinner: Thai salad (322 calories)
Total: 540 calories

Meal Plan 3:

Breakfast: 1 sliced apple and 1 sliced mangoes with 1 small hardboiled egg (223 calories)
Lunch: mushroom stroganoff (90 calories)
Dinner: Tuna, beans, and garlic salad (267 calories)
Total: 580 calories

Meal Plan 4:

Breakfast: 1small hardboiled egg, 3 pieces of low-fat ham and 1 tangerine (140 calories)
Lunch: asparagus with garlic-mayo dip (88 calories)
Dinner: pizza topped with vegetables (358 calories)
Total: 586 calories